ZELANDA DOWELL

FOOD RX

Cocoa Butter Blend for Healthy Nourished Skin

Pink Lemonade Publishing

CONTENTS

CONTENTS

FOOD RX:

Cocoa Butter Blend
for Healthy Nourished Skin

Zelanda Dowell

COPYRIGHT

———————————

To request permissions, contact the publisher at: Pinklemonadepublishing@gmail.com

ISBN Paperback: 978-1-7367299-1-5
ISBN eBook: 978-1-7367299-0-8

Printed by Ingram Spark
Pink Lemonade Publishing LLC
P.O. Box 96
Bloomfield Hills, MI.

FOOD RX

48304 USA

Pinklemonadepublishing.com

DEDICATION

To my children,
whom I want to live and model a healthier life for.

PREFACE

Hello there!

Maybe you're interested in this book because natural skincare excites your interest. Perhaps you want to start a natural skincare business or make handmade gifts. Are you curious? Do you have dry skin that never seems to get better?

No matter why you are reading this book, I'm sure you'll learn something about natural skincare regimens and how they affect our health.

I am writing this book to share what I've learned, my experiences, health benefits, and even a few words from people I've given my cocoa butter blend.

I hope you truly enjoy this book, the cocoa butter blend, and the praise you'll receive from your partakers; believe me, it's coming!

Thank you for purchasing and reading my book.

Share this book with someone who you think would love it, or make use of some skin-nourishing knowledge!

Cheers to healthy skin!
Zelanda Dowell

THE NECESSITY

"Necessity is the mother of invention" - Plato

Have you ever applied lotion to dry skin, just to look down in five minutes or so, and your skin is dry again? Yep! I feel your pain.

Sure, many people have dry skin, but lotion should fix that, right? WRONG.

Most lotions contain alcohol, which is useful for preserving but is drying to your skin. Most lotion/cream contain fragrances, which smell great but are also drying and irritating to your skin.

I have the same dehydrated skin that my Mom had. My skin looks like a carbon copy of hers.

"Drink more water," my Dad encourages. Drinking water does help with overall hydration, yet my dry skin remains after drinking way more water than usual.

"Try my oatmeal lotion in there on the dresser. That's all I use." My grandma instructed. I tried the lotion for a while; applied it the way she does too. Yet the skin on my body still craved more, while the skin on my face broke out in hives.

"Ma! My skin is so dry, and I'm allergic to almost everything!" I cried out to my Mom, depleted.

"Breathe. You're a visionary. You'll figure this out." She said encouragingly. "And when you figure it out, whatever *it* is, share it with your mama!" She laughed. My Mom always had a way of breathing peace onto me, then sealing the deal with laughter.

THE CLASSIC 100% COCOA BUTTER STICK

I am thankful that I can now say my youngest daughter *had* terrible eczema break-outs. My daughter has eczema, and I have eczema and seborrheic dermatitis. My Mom had eczema and seborrheic dermatitis. You get the point; dry skin runs in the family.

When I started carrying a purse in elementary school, my grandma would make me take a cocoa butter stick. You know the yellow tubes packed with solid 100% pure cocoa butter that are a pain-in-the-you-know-what to use when it gets low? Yep. My grandma made sure I had plenty.

That cocoa butter did wonders for my skin! I'd apply it anywhere that was dry—my hands, face, hand, lips, elbows, knees, and more. Cocoa butter is thick, fatty, and oh so moisturizing! It soothes skin like no other, not to mention I love smelling like chocolate!

Like many things that I loved, the classic yellow tube of 100% cocoa butter, I had an equal amount of pet peeves as well. The cocoa butter packaging makes it travel-ready, yet it's hard to apply when the tube gets low. Cocoa butter packed in the travel-sized tube is hard to apply to larger areas of the body.

Let's talk about some of the pros and cons of using cocoa butter!

Cocoa Butter's Pros

- Good for skin hydration and elasticity
- Creates a protective layer on the skin to hold moisture in
- Improves blood flow
- Protects skin from harmful UV rays
- Slows aging
- Reduces scars, wrinkles, and other marks
- Heals rashes from eczema and dermatitis
- Could prevent/treat skin diseases
- Edible
- Plant-based fat
- High in fatty acid

Cocoa Butter's Cons

- Cocoa butter can cause an allergic reaction for

some, although allergies to the cocoa bean are rare.
· Cocoa butter is considered comedogenic and can clog facial pores.

Cocoa Butter's Make-up

· Arachidic acid: promotes and repairs
· Linoleic acid: strengthens skin natural protective barrier, moisturizing, and healing
· Oleic acid: wound recovery and permeability enhancing
· Palmitic acid: emollient, skin softener, and moisture retainer
· Stearic acid: cleans pores and locks in moisture

Whew! With a line-up like that, no wonder many people swear by cocoa butter.

COCONUT OIL

One of nature's wonders

Almost six years ago, my youngest daughter was born with eczema. Her pediatrician at the time prescribed her medicated cream intended for use once daily.

Watching my baby scratch her skin raw and hearing her cry from the itching is something that bothers me. I often kept the cream at the ready to slather her skin. Day after day, I applied the cream to her skin, but one day I forgot; and I realized something strange.

In a little over 24 hours, her skin went from clear and smooth to itchy, bumpy, and inflamed! I knew something wasn't right.

I called the doctor's office to hear, "That is normal. Keep using the cream as directed."

I didn't accept that as an answer. Yes, that reaction is known to that medication, but that shouldn't be normal for healthy skin. When the doctor prescribed the cream, I believed that this cream would make her skin healthy, but it only masked the symptoms.

This incident opened my mind; I wanted to know why her skin reacted negatively so quickly. After that tube was gone, I promised myself I wasn't using steroid medicated cream on my baby's skin anymore.

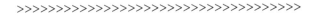

I've done extensive medical research. I've read page after page of countless medical books. I went to college for medical assisting as a teenager, but I didn't learn much about natural medicine. For the last six to seven years, I've been studying natural healing and herbology.

I've learned that the skin can become reliant on steroid creams; my daughter's skin had done just that.

Now that I was down to her last few applications, I had a few natural skincare ideas that I wanted to try on her. On a grocery store trip, I grabbed a small jar of organic unrefined virgin cold-pressed coconut oil. From my internet research, coconut oil for skin can be a hit for some and a miss for others. In my Natural Healing course, it's a hit. So, I decided to grab it.

After a warm bath before bed, I rubbed my baby down

from head to toe in coconut oil. (Coconut oil is solid in temperatures below seventy-eight degrees Fahrenheit.) My baby slept great! She went to sleep quickly, and she stayed asleep without waking up to scratch.

From that day on, I will always use natural materials on her skin. Now, almost six years later, she's had two eczema flare-ups, and the two flares that she's had so far were minor. And the best part? No steroid cream was involved.

All-natural organic unrefined cold-pressed virgin coconut oil did that for her! Coconut oil is better for your overall skin health than steroid creams or prescriptions meant to mask the symptoms. Coconut oil gives skin the moisture it needs while attacking the problem's primary source, not the aftermath.

100% Coconut Oil

Coconut Oil's Pros

- A plant-based fat (almost 100% fat)
- High in vitamin E
- Edible
- It kills bacteria and fungi
- Reduces inflammation
- Reduces skin pain from psoriasis, contact dermatitis, and eczema

- Treats acne
- Promotes hydration
- Treats eczema/dry skin
- Aids in wound/burn healing
- Increases collagen levels
- High in antioxidants (reduces free radicals)

Coconut Oil's Cons

- May cause allergic reactions in some people
- May clog pores in some people with oily/sensitive skin

Coconut Oil's Make-up

- Saturated fat: stops dry skin, inflammation, and premature aging
- Medium-chain fatty acids: antimicrobial properties that prevent harmful microorganisms that cause things like athlete's foot and cellulitis
- Lauric acid: antibacterial properties that prevent acne
- Myristic acid: promotes skin hydration and a youthful appearance
- Caprylic acid: effectively treats acne
- Palmitic acid: emollient, skin softener, and moister retainer
- Capric acid: nourishes problematic/ acne-prone skin

- Oleic acid: wound healing and permeability enhancing
- Linoleic acid: strengthens skin natural protective barrier, moisturizing, and healing
- Stearic acid: cleans pores and locks in moisture

SWEET ALMOND OIL

When it comes to the cocoa butter blend that has allowed me to stop buying lotion (or any skin moisturizer, for that matter), I'd say without hesitation; this recipe/product has worked wonders for my family and those I have given it to! This cocoa butter blend contains all-natural ingredients, high-quality materials and is nourishing to the skin.

We have talked about the first part of this recipe: organic unrefined cold-pressed virgin coconut oil, which is super hydrating, light, and antibacterial. Coconut oil packs a highly nutritious punch.

The second part of the recipe is organic 100% pure cocoa butter. The cocoa butter is moisturizing, protective, and heavier, which helps to solidify this blend.

The third and final part of this recipe is interchangeable with many different oils, which I will explain later, but now I'll focus on my favorite two: almond oil and olive oil. Let's take a look at almond oil.

Almond oil reminds me of coconut oil in a few ways:

- Almond oil is light oil.
- Almond oil is incredibly hydrating and absorbs quickly into the skin.
- Almond oil is anti-inflammatory.

Almond oil is excellent to add to your skincare routine because it is a light moisturizer and is also non-comedogenic, which means it won't clog your pores. Look at the breakdown of almond health facts below!

Almond Oil's Pros

- Good as a skin moisturizer
- Improves acne
- Can prevent and/or reduce stretch marks
- Helps reverse damage from the sun
- Can improve complexion and skin tone
- Treats dry skin conditions like psoriasis and eczema
- Reduces under-eye circles and puffy eyes
- Reduces the appearance of scars and stretch marks

Almond Oil's Cons

- If you have an almond allergy, using almond oil could cause an allergic reaction

Almond's Make-up

- Oleic acid: promotes and repairs
- Linoleic acid: strengthens skin natural protective barrier, moisturizing, and healing
- Palmitic acid: emollient, skin softener, and moisture retainer
- Stearic acid: cleans pores and locks in moisture
- Arachidic acid: promotes and repairs

Almond oil! Where have you been my whole life?

Suppose you have an allergy to tree nuts (even if it is minor). In that case, you'll want to refrain from using almond oil in this recipe, as repeatedly exposing yourself to something you are allergic to can make your allergy to that item worse over time. Keep reading for another option.

EXTRA VIRGIN OLIVE OIL

My third favorite ingredient that I use in my batches of cocoa butter blend is organic extra virgin olive oil.

I love cooking; I'm a food blogger/author and a hard-core foodie, so olive oil is always something I have.

The addition of olive oil in this cocoa butter blend makes a luxurious plant-based butter-like moisturizer that feels heavenly gliding onto your skin. A nice hot shower and a jar of cocoa butter blend are genuinely part of my self-love regimen.

Now, putting all lux feels aside, many of us have olive oil in our pantries right now; why not use it as part of our skincare routines as well? Olive oil moisturizes, is high in antioxidants, kills acne-causing bacteria, and can even work to kill cancer-causing cells! Who knew all these health benefits could come with the oil pressed from an olive?

Just as olive oil has many great qualities, it also can

have some drawbacks. Olive oil is heavy oil and can be comedogenic. Using too much olive oil on your face can have the opposite effect and trap bacteria, which can cause acne break-outs in people with sensitive skin.

Let's check out the health benefits of olive oil.

Olive Oil's Pros

- Good for moisturizing
- Fighting bacteria decreasing acne
- Rich in vitamins A,D,K and E
- Prevents cancer caused by harmful UV rays
- Slows aging
- Reduces scars, wrinkles, and other marks
- Heals rashes from eczema and dermatitis
- Could prevent/treat skin diseases
- Edible
- Plant-based fat
- High in fatty acid

Olive Oil's Cons

- Olive oil is a heavy oil; putting too much on the skin can do the opposite and trap bacteria/clog pores, causing acne and/or other skin issues.

Olive Oil's Make-up

- Palmitic acid: emollient, skin softener, and moister retainer
- Palmitoleic acid: treats skin hyperpigmentation and promotes wound healing
- Stearic acid: cleans pores and locks in moisture
- Oleic acid: wound recovery and permeability enhancing
- Linoleic acid: strengthens skin natural protective barrier, moisturizing, and healing
- Myristic acid: keeps skin hydrated and youthful

So far, we've covered what makes these individual oils great on their own; let's summarize their prowess when blended.

LET'S SUMMERIZE

· Coconut oil. Cocoa butter and almond oil (or olive oil) make up this fragrant cocoa butter blend.
· It is made of all-natural plant-based fats to help treat dry skin, eczema, other skin sensitivities/issues or be used as a natural alternative to traditional lotion/moisturizers.
· When it comes to eczema treatments, there are no absolutes. This recipe may be great for someone, while it can be the opposite for another. Always preform a spot check when trying out a new product on your skin.
· This recipe thrives in versatility! You can change the recipe/ingredients as you see fit for you and your family using the recipe guidelines provided!

ADDITIONAL INFO

· According to the FDA, coconuts are considered tree nuts, yet they aren't botanical nuts. They are considered fruits. Coconut allergies are rarer than other "tree nuts." Most people who are allergic to tree nuts can safely eat coconuts, while some people can't. To be sure, check with your allergist/doctor if you have a tree nut allergy to be sure you can safely use coconut oil.

- Cocoa butter comes from the cocoa bean, which also grows on trees. Allergies to cocoa butter are infrequent, but if you question this item's safety, check with your allergist/doctor.
- If you have sensitive skin (like me) and you're worried about how your skin will do with a new product, do a patch test. Try applying cocoa butter blend on an area of skin on the body about two inches square. Watch for 24-48 hours to see any changes. If no negative changes occur, go on to use as usual.
- When making batches of cocoa butter for my home, I always buy certified organic food-grade oils. Certified organic products promise to have no chemicals or anything non-organic included
- I like to buy food-grade items because food-grade items are kept cleaner and are okay to eat. I often use cocoa butter blend on my lips, so food-grade items are essential to me. (Whatever someone applies to the lips can unintentionally end up in the stomach in trace amounts.)
- I store my homemade cocoa butter blend in short wide glass mason jars. Glass is a lovely natural-preserving container! Glass keeps its contents fresher longer without leaching harmful chemicals into

your products over time. Oh, and glass mason jars are reusable (no matter the brand), dishwasher safe, microwave safe, and freezer safe (double check on the jar label).

· I like to use short wide mouth glass mason jars because they're easier to get your fingers and hand into.

COCOA BUTTER BLEND
VISUAL RECIPE

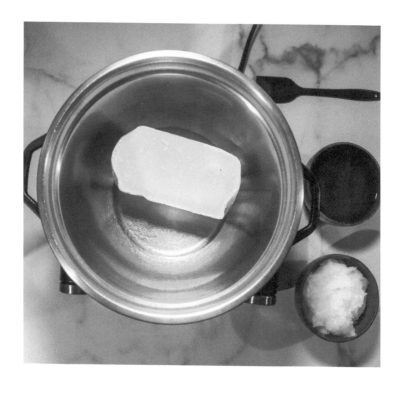

First, make the Bain Marie or double boiler to melt
and mix oils.

MELT

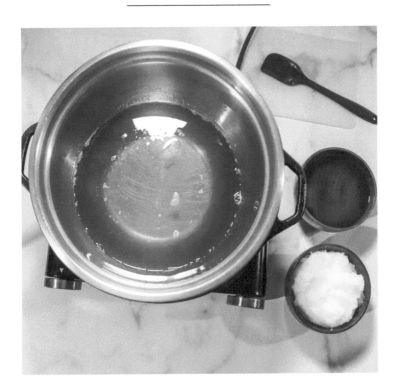

Melt solid cocoa butter down to liquid.

ADD COCONUT OIL

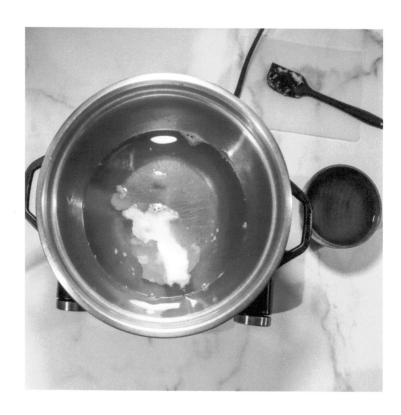

Add coconut oil, gently stirring to encourage melt-ing.

ADD OLIVE OIL

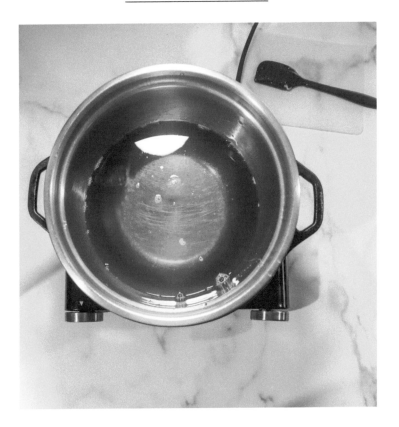

Add olive oil and gently stir, blending oils.

SPOON

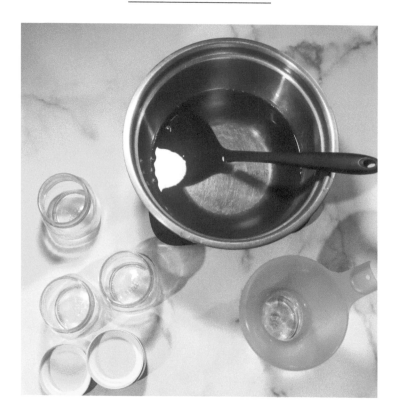

If you are making the easiest cocoa butter blend, spoon hot oils into clean glass jars, cool on the counter for about an hour, then leave to harden in the fridge overnight.

COOL

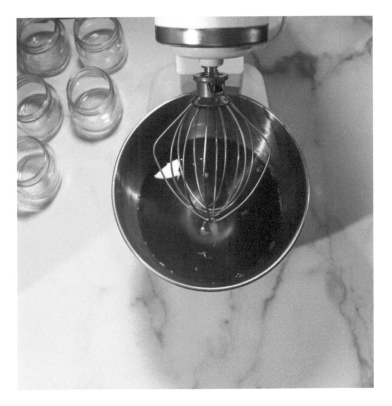

If you're making whipped cocoa butter, cool oils in the freezer and attach wire whisk attachment preparing to whip.

WHIP

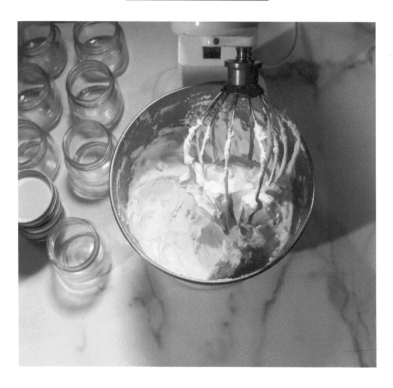

After oils are cooled, whip on medium speed until
stiff peaks form.

STIR

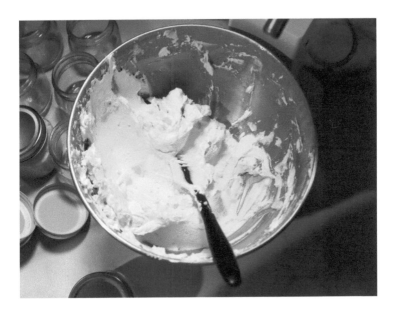

Stir whipped cocoa butter to check for even mixing.

STORE

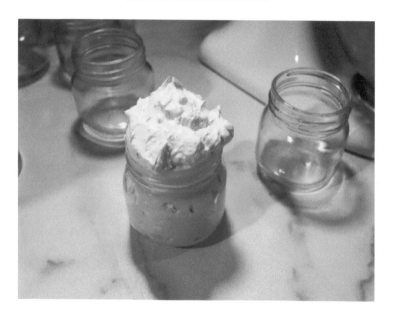

Spoon whipped cocoa butter in clean jars to sit on the counter top overnight.

COCOA BUTTER BLEND RECIPE

───────────────

A naturally fragrant blend that nourishes and hydrates skin without any harsh artificial ingredients!

- Makes: Four to Five 8 Ounce Jars
- Takes: 15-45 minutes depending on the type you choose to make.
- Difficulty: Easy

Ingredients

- 1 Pound Organic Raw Unrefined Cocoa Butter
- 8 Ounces Organic Unrefined Cold-pressed Virgin Coconut Oil
- 8 Ounces Organic Extra Virgin Olive Oil See recipe notes for oil alternatives.

Instructions

1. In a Bain Marie or double boiler, start boiling water

over high heat. Once the water is boiling, turn down to medium heat.

2. Add cocoa butter to top boiler (making sure it melts, but stays dry).

3. When the cocoa butter is completely melted, add coconut oil.

4. Stir gently until coconut oil melts completely.

5. Add olive oil.

6. Stir gently for 30 second to 1 minute to blend oils.

7. Remove from heat, then spoon melted oil blend into glass jars to store.

8. Let glass jars cool on the counter for about an hour.

9. To get oils to firm up, leave them on the counter undisturbed until they are solid (a day or more depending on the temperature of your home). To firm up quicker, put jars in the fridge over night or 8 plus hours.

10. After sitting, open a jar to check if cocoa butter blend has completely firmed up. If not, leave on the counter or in the fridge another 8 hours.

11. Use cocoa butter blend like you would any lotion or body butter.

12. Enjoy your new favorite handmade skincare item!

Recipe Notes

- If you don't have a Bain Marie, you can make one with a sauce pot and a slightly bigger stainless steel mixing bowl! Fill the sauce pot 2/3 full with water, then set large stainless steel mixing bowl on top. Make sure the bowl is small enough to set on top of the sauce pot with some of the bowl resting in the pot, but big enough that the bowl won't move around while the water is boiling.

· Melting oils in the microwave works great too! Add the cocoa butter into a large microwavable bowl or a large microwave safe glass measuring cup. (I use an 8 cup Pyrex measuring cup.) Microwave for 2 minutes, stir, then microwave for 30-second intervals until cocoa butter is fully melted. Remove melted cocoa butter from microwave and add coconut oil then olive oil. The coconut oil will melt from residual heat, no need to microwave more. Follow steps 7 through 12 to complete cocoa butter blend.

· When I make Cocoa Butter Blend for my home, I always use organic food-grade ingredients. Food-grade or organic ingredients are not necessary, but healthier.

· Great oil substitutions for extra virgin olive oil are sweet almond oil, avocado oil, grapeseed oil, jojoba oil, argan oil, rosehip oil, and apricot kernel oil.

· If you prefer a whipped butter instead of a more solid one, follow instructions 1-7 except don't pour hot oils in jars. Leave hot oils in a large mixing bowl or a stand mixer bowl, putting the oils in the freezer for 20-30 minutes. With a whisk attachment, beat oil until it turns white, and stiff peaks form. Spoon into clean glass jars, apply lid, and let whipped cocoa butter blend rest/cool on the counter overnight.

· Be creative! This cocoa butter blend can be kept in other containers like plastic or tin. I use glass because it's free from harsh chemicals that could leach into the finished product and it's reusable.

REFERENCES

1. Rachael Link MS RD, 2017, Healthline, www.healthline.com/nutrition/coconut-oil-and-skin#TOC_TITLE_HDR_2
2. 2020, Fleur & Bee fleurandbee.com/blogs/news/coconut-oil-for-skin
3. Danielle Dresden, 2020, Medical News Today www.medicalnewstoday.com/articles/coconut-oil-good-for-skin
4. Laurene Boateng, Richard Asong, William B. Owusu, Matilda Steiner-Asiedu, 2016, Ghana Medical Journal www.ncbi.nlm.nih.gov/pmc/articles/PMC5044790/#:~:text=Co-conut%20oil%20is%20com-posed%20of,-18%3A2%20linoleic%20acid.
5. Grace Gallagher, 2019, Healthline ,www.health-line.com/health/beauty-skin-care/almond-oil-for-face#benefits
6. Lindsay Curtis, 2020, Very Well Health, www.very-wellhealth.com/almond-oil-for-skin-5083921
7. Lowri Daniels, 2020, Medical News Today,

www.medicalnewstoday.com/articles/almond-oil-for-skin

8. Z Shi,Q Fu,B Chen,S Xu,1999, National Library of Medicine,://pubmed.ncbi.nlm.nih.gov/12552899/

9. Gabriel D. Fernandes, Raquel B. Gómez-Coca, María del Carmen Pérez-Camino, Wenceslao Moreda, and Daniel Barrera-Arellano, 2017 Hindawi Journal of Medicine   www.hindawi.com/journals/jchem/2017/2609549/

10. ChaunieBrusie,2018,   Healthline,   www.health-line.com/health/olive-oil-benefits-face#:~:text=It%20moisturizes%20and%20fights%2

11. Jayne Leonard, 2018, Medical News Today ://www.medicalnewstoday.com/articles/321246

12. Carrie Madormo RN, MPH, 2021, Very Well Health://www.verywellhealth.com/olive-oil-skin-benefits-5095861

13. Nicole Blades, 2019, Good House Keeping, www.goodhousekeeping.com/beauty/anti-aging/a28775913/olive-oil-for-skin/

14. Wikipedia en.m.wikipedia.org/wiki/Olive_oil

15. Stephanie Watson, 2017, Healthline www.health-line.com/health/beauty-skin-care/cocoa-butter-benefits#benefits

16. Jen Adkins & Carolyn Hanson, 2019, Byrdie https://www.byrdie.com/the-benefits-of-cocoa-butter-for-your-skin-3013590

17. Aaron Mandola, 2019, Medical News Today www.medicalnewstoday.com/articles/325227

18. 2020,Web MD, www.webmd.com/diet/health-ben-efits-cocoa-butter
19. Wikipedia en.m.wikipedia.org/wiki/Cocoa_butter
20. Kristin Collins Jackson, 2016, Bustle, www.bustle.com/articles/164350-7-lightweight-face-oils-that-wont-leave-your-skin-feeling-greasy-photos

THANK YOU FROM THE BOTTOM OF MY HEART!

_____

Thank you for reading Food Rx: Cocoa Butter Blend for Healthy Nourished Skin! I hope that you enjoyed this book and that you've learned enough to start your natural skincare journey, or better yet, learn to use food for medicine!

Please share this book with someone who you think would make great use of it!

Sending love from my kitchen to yours!
-Zelanda Dowell

Website: www.zelandaskitchen.com
Social Media: www.lnk.bio/zelandaskitchen
Email: Zelandaskitchen@gmail.com

CPSIA information can be obtained
at www.ICGtesting.com
Printed in the USA
LVHW072132220921
698455LV00001B/5